The Truth About Real Beauty

Just **STOP** THE **LIES!**

SECRETS THE BEAUTY INDUSTRY DOESN'T WANT YOU TO KNOW

By: The Authority in Beauty

David Pollock

JUST STOP THE LIES!

Designer: Samantha Watson

Editors: Dawn Davis, Melissa Elbrand, Corain Cash, Megan McKenzie, Samantha Watson, William Rodriguez

Printed and bound in the United States of America
Fourth printing, July 2012

Library of Congress Control Number: 2010910774
ISBN-10 098289340X
ISBN-13 9780982893401

Just Ask David, LLC.
1700 NW 65th Avenue North - #13
Plantation, FL 33313 USA
Visit our Website at www.JustAskDavid.com
Email: david@justaskdavid.com

Contents

Introduction   V

Chapter 1

The Naked Truth About Beauty   1

Chapter 2

Beauty From Within   31

Chapter 3

The Truth About What's Inside   48

Chapter 4

Is Your Skin Cream Aging You?   80

Chapter 5

Does Your Skin Cream Cause Cancer?   92

Conclusion   102

For Every Woman

Introduction

I am often asked, what made you decide to pursue a career in the cosmetics industry? Simple. There are two key factors that influenced my decision.

First, I have three sisters. Growing up, I watched them use every different cosmetic product imaginable. They are, all three, beautiful ladies, but each of them still carried out daily regimens to maintain their beauty, and to highlight features and disguise whatever imperfections they thought they had.

Second, there are few industries that can remain steady in a difficult economy. No matter what a woman's budget, she is going to find a way to purchase whatever she needs to maintain her appearance.

It was easy to realize that this would be an industry that could only grow. Even today, I am still amazed at the amount of products women store in their bathroom drawers and under the counters - even similar products from different brands. Women will try almost anything to look and feel better about themselves.

So, why become the authority in beauty? As my grandfather taught me as a young boy, "Anything worth doing, is worth doing right." So I have spent the last twenty some-odd years learning everything I can and building my name in the industry.

Introduction

Throughout my career, I have developed products for some of the most prestigious names in the beauty industry. (I have to admit, it is exciting to walk through a store and see people looking at a product you created.) My experience in research and development is augmented by my experience in marketing and management as former Vice President at the Home Shopping Network, Founder of Clinical Results development laboratory, CEO of Hydron Technologies, and Senior Executive with the Fuller Brush Company.

Along the way, I have created several new skin care technologies, been a keynote speaker at various national conferences, written numerous articles for trade and consumer publications, and was recently named one of the "20 to Know" in 2010 by Global Cosmetics Industry (GCI) magazine.

Today, I sit on the board of several skin care companies and am the publisher of an online magazine called www.JustAskDavid.com.

So why write this book? Why disclose secrets of the beauty industry? Won't I upset some of the companies that I have worked with?

Simple. I have spent my career developing state-of-the-art products. While some companies really do care about the quality of the product and the results the consumer will experience, there are a number of companies that will simply push the envelope in trying to cut costs, failing to keep the promises made to the consumer.

Introduction

I remember once developing a line of products for a brand (which shall remain nameless) that I won't name. I was brought on a sales call to meet with the buyer of a large retailer, so I could answer any technical questions. I explained how this was a unique product with a high level of actives, moderately priced, clinically proven - and guaranteed to deliver results. The buyer cut the conversation short and said, "Mama doesn't know. Sprinkle in the active, drop the price to $2.99 and I'll buy truckloads of it." I was speechless. I was insulted. Shame on that buyer. Shame on the retailer that would allow this type of practice to take place.

Then it hit me - I realized then that "Mama" should know! The question was how to tell her.

Today, I have become a consumer advocate, focused on bringing a change to the beauty industry. My goal is to inform the consumer about the secrets of the beauty industry - from the definition of true beauty to the damage caused by certain ingredients found in products we use every day.

To achieve my goal, I decided to write a book. I knew it had to be informative, yet fun to read. When you read the book, you will see the real me. You will see my passion to deliver my message, as well as the humor and fun I try to put in to life everyday!

My goal is simple. I want to empower you to realize your true beauty, to understand what is really in products you use every day, and how some skin creams may actually be aging you - or even worse, contain ingredients that can cause cancer!

I have broken it down into five core areas:

- The Naked Truth About Beauty
  Empowers women to realize their true beauty
- Beauty From Within
  Explains the effects various foods have on our skin
- The Truth About What's Inside
  Uncovers tricks of the industry - including the truth behind cosmetic claims
- Is Your Skin Cream Aging You?
  Exposes how traditional skin creams can actually be damaging and aging your skin
- Does Your Skin Cream Cause Cancer?
  Reveals ingredients that can be dangerous and new technologies that provide a safe solution

With this book, "Mama" can know and make an educated decision - and "Mama" can vote with her pocketbook.

Brands, Retailers - get ready! Just Stop the Lies! The TRUTH is out! Consumers are becoming aware. Consumers are demanding safe products that deliver. **It's time to adapt or become extinct!**

~ Chapter One ~

The Naked Truth About Beauty

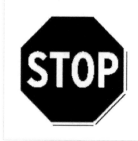

STOP! STOP! STOP!
STOP the media! STOP the beauty industry!
STOP THE LIES!

Forget everything you've been told to believe what beauty is. The truth is, what you have been taught is WRONG!

The fashion and beauty industries want to sell you magazines and products. How? Obviously, *not* by telling you that you're beautiful and perfect the way you are. Rather, they make their money by being negative and telling you that you have a lot to change to look beautiful – that's what sells more magazines and more beauty products.

The thousands of articles and beauty advertisements that bombard you set a standard of beauty that no person can achieve. By feeding off women's insecurities about the natural aging process, the beauty industry encourages women to spend billions of dollars in a futile attempt to attain unnatural and everlasting youth. The models pictured in these advertisements are often very young, may have had cosmetic treatments or even plastic surgery and have had professional hair stylists and professional makeup artists prepare them for the photo shoot.

And yet, many of the photos are *still* air-brushed to perfection. What? That's right, they are air-brushed - *where imperfections are removed or touched up using computer software.* And this is the image and standard you are told to strive for.

The truth is that models are fortunate enough to have a professional do their hair and make-up, but nobody - including models - can actually achieve the false image portrayed in advertising.

Are you kidding me? Sadly, no. The beauty industry should be about enhancing each individual woman's beauty, not creating a market where women will stop at no cost in a desperate attempt to conform to an artificial and idealized image of beauty. Instead, media and advertising by the beauty industry have successfully destroyed the self-esteem of many women, leading to an obsession with beauty and perfection. From dieting to applying makeup, girls learn at young ages how to alter themselves to meet this idealized image of beauty – often leading to unhealthy outcomes, both physical and mental.

As the authority in beauty, I see a lot. But I think the most eye-opening example of this obsession to me was at a red carpet event in New York. I had just helped launch a new anti-wrinkle skin care technology. I met numerous women of all ages (*HINT: Now you know why I got into the beauty industry – LOL!*), but one girl stood out. Not because of her beauty, but because of our conversation. She was striking, but obviously young. She asked me how to get rid of a wrinkle that was starting to form by her eyes. I looked and laughed.

I didn't see any wrinkles – not one. But she insisted that one was starting to form. I tried to explain to her how striking she was and how when she walked over, every guy's head turned. She laughed and said that wasn't her worry, she was a cover model. She explained that the trend is to use younger models and just one small wrinkle could end her career.

Pause here for a second. I'll bet you are thinking the same thing I was. She was a model that had appeared on the covers of magazines. How could she be concerned about her appearance? What could I possibly say? Actually, a lot.... So, I opened my big mouth and asked, "Why are we even having this conversation? You are the unrealistic image the beauty industry is telling women they should look like!"

Okay, I know what to do...I will write a book and scream it to the world: The fashion and beauty industry are a business, a business generating billions of dollars a year – and all the while they are stealing your money and self-esteem. STOP IT, STOP IT, STOP IT – Shame on them!

Don't get me wrong, I am not saying that you should stop caring about how you dress, stop taking care of your skin, or stop using make-up. What I am saying is that the beauty industry's definition of beauty is wrong and they are doing more harm than good with the messages they are delivering. I want to change that. I want you to realize that YOU are beautiful...just as you are!

Let me say that again, YOU ARE BEAUTIFUL – JUST AS YOU ARE!

Of course, we all have things we are concerned about and want to change. The key is to minimize or forget about your imperfections and highlight your best features – this starts on the inside with your self confidence. Your smile, your eyes say it all!

Defining Beauty

The reason I started in this industry is simple. Unlike other industries, I knew that the beauty industry would only continue to grow in any economy. Good times or bad, the industry will be one of the few that will continue to see growth. Why? Because, no woman I have ever met is happy with her appearance. That's right, across the vast spectrum of women, from cover models to the girls next door, I have never met a woman that sees herself as beautiful.

Well, let me ask you – do you feel beautiful just as you are? Or do you have a list of things you want to change? While I plan to tell you things you can do to help you achieve your beauty goals, my real goal is to help you appreciate you...just as you are!

I have a close friend that is absolutely beautiful, inside and out. One trait that may even enhance her overall beauty is that she has never let her physical beauty go to her head. Well, one day I, sadly, found out why. She really never saw it in herself. One day, back in college, she called me in tears. The university had picked 12 girls, including her, to be in the upcoming year's calendar. I was excited for her and couldn't figure out why she was crying, so she finally explained, "They picked eleven beautiful girls and one to make fun of." I laughed for a second, until I realized she actually believed what she was saying. Now, when I look back on that phone call, I get teary-eyed. Why would someone have such doubt about themselves? What would it be like to feel that way? More importantly, what could I do to help her see her beauty and how the world saw her – and not just her physical beauty, but the overall person, inside and out?

In a culture of ideals and perfect images, I see women go to great lengths to alter their appearances, yet remain dissatisfied and continue to experience feelings of being unattractive. Every woman – that's right, every woman that I have ever met – has at least one item they want to change. Think for a moment. If you could, what would you change about yourself?

Be prepared. I am going to help you achieve *real* beauty and feel confident about yourself. Okay, do me a favor. Walk over to the mirror and look for a moment. Ready? Stare deep. You know what? I see it! I see it! I see a beautiful woman staring back at you. That's right. Beautiful. And you are very lucky! And any significant other you choose to let into your life is even luckier!

I have to ask, "Do you see it?" Because, if you hesitate to scream, "I SEE IT!" I want to share with you what I have learned from twenty years in the beauty industry. By the end of this book, I am going to help you be able to scream "I SEE IT!"

You see, there are two truths to begin with when discussing beauty:

The first is that all women are similar, in the sense that every woman desires to be seen as beautiful. The problem is that the beauty industry paints an unachievable, distorted image of what it means to be attractive – leaving women confused about how to precisely define beauty.

Consider, for a moment, that if I were to create a list of the items that are involved in the beauty process, would it truly reflect the perfect woman? Of course not. The perfect woman is you, just as you are. Can you create a regimen to help you focus on your attributes, maybe improve a few things you consider "imperfections," and help you feel better about your true beauty? Yes, and that is what I want to accomplish here with this book.

The beauty industry wants you to believe that a woman must not only have long hair, but hair which exudes volume and movement. Her body must be lean, toned and never reveal a hint of cellulite. Her breasts must be perky and full and more than likely augmented to match her derriere, which is firm, elevated and looks great in a mini skirt. Let's not forget the toned, tanned (albeit sprayed on) legs that are wearing a pair of stilettos to emphasize the beauty of her calves. Her hip hugger jeans look amazing resting on her six pack abs. The skin on her body is velvety smooth and alluring. The skin on her face is poreless, lineless, and may not have much movement thanks to Botox®, Restylane® or even a face lift. Her eyes will never droop and her under-eye bags have been eliminated. What about those voluptuous lips, which protect the most perfect white-as-snow teeth?

Who is this woman? This is the woman who has been created by the media and the woman who has defined this century's idea of what is beautiful. Is this really beauty?

When asking many of my female friends and acquaintances, the consensus is that women feel they are judged primarily by outward appearance. Never before has there been such scrutiny regarding the ideal image of beauty, and, unfortunately, with today's definition of beauty, it takes more than natural beauty to be considered ravishing.

Magazine articles, photographs, and advertisements all bombard us with the message that this is what it takes to be beautiful, and that, with enough time, money, and products, anyone can look like a model. What I think is even worse is that the styles and images continually change, creating an unachievable, moving target. Why? The answer, of course, is to keep us buying. Because after all, if you want to achieve the perfect image, you will buy more magazines and more products that target every aspect of your appearance, from head to toe.

The media leads women to believe that beauty is defined as being free of imperfection. However, isn't nature, itself, imperfect – yet also beautiful? The truth is that beauty is a subjective concept, one which cannot be objectified and defined by a narrow set of qualities or features. This can clearly be seen when examining the chasms that exist in the definitions of beauty across cultures and regions throughout the world. While a full and voluptuous body is considered beautiful in Ghana, by contrast, a petite frame defines beauty in the Japanese culture. These variances in the definitions of beauty across cultures highlight the truth that beauty is subjective and defined by individuals; there is no universal standard. In the end, an individual's definition of beauty is influenced by many factors, including culture, geography, personal opinion, and experiences - and, of course, media exposure. The bottom line is that individuals have long relied on external comparisons, validation, and confirmation to tell them what beautiful looks like.

So, what happens if you are actually human, normal and possibly overweight, with thinning hair and wrinkles on your face? Does this mean that you are not considered attractive? Are we *that* shallow? Do we really believe that "beauty is skin deep"? Well, yes, unfortunately, most people do believe this - and, more importantly, most women believe this about themselves...until now! I am here to change that!

Don't misunderstand, every woman wants to look her best - and there is nothing wrong with the desire to enhance your appearance. Perhaps you may choose a great pair of shoes or a fashion accessory that accentuates your best feature. But do we really have to buy in to the message that physical allure is all a woman has to offer? Is beauty *actually* just skin deep? I say "NO WAY! ABSOLUTELY NOT!" - which brings me to the second truth.

The second truth is that *real* beauty is you. That's right, there is no reason to obsess over little imperfections, when physical perfection is not achievable – there is no such thing as physical perfection. Actually, it should not even be desired, because the real beauty is you – YOU, JUST AS YOU ARE!

It is precisely the little things that make us unique and attractive to others. So, while the shape of our nose, the size of our ears, the number of freckles, or the thickness of our eyebrows may be seen by some as imperfections, they are really attributes that makes us different, unique... enchanting. Picture the unique "flaws" that made Marilyn Monroe, Cindy Crawford, or Julia Roberts actually stand apart from the crowd. We should embrace the characteristics that make us different and special.

Even with all of the cultural influences being thrust upon us, each individual defines beauty differently, and it is for this reason that each and every woman must look within herself to appreciate both her "perfections" and imperfections as contributions to the beautiful and unique expression of herself!

That's right. Real beauty is not a perfect outer image, but rather the combination of outer beauty and inner beauty – imperfections and all!

In the end, the struggle to be beautiful is really all about sex appeal and the search for validation of our beauty and attractiveness to the opposite sex. By the way, this goes for men, too, not just women. We all have heard the old adage that beauty is in the eye of the beholder. Well, it really is – everyone looks for something different. Here's an example of what I mean: My best friend and I have known each other for over 28 years (*Wow, he must be old! LOL*). One reason we have remained such good friends is that we have never pursued the same girl or let a girl come between us. How could that be? The answer is simple and proves my point. No matter how similar we are, we both define beauty differently. We discovered this early on in our friendship.

One day we were at our favorite restaurant having lunch, when two girls walked in and sat down across the room. Throughout our meal, we both kept commenting on how good-looking one of the girls was. We each challenged the other to go talk to her, but were both too shy to actually say anything. Anyway, at one point toward the end of the meal, I commented on what a knock-out the brunette was and how much she looked to be my type. After my friend got done chuckling, he asked, "What are you talking about? Her? She isn't that good looking – it's her friend, the blonde, I've been talking about." After I almost choked on my food, I had to ask him, "What are you talking about? The blonde has nothing on her friend the brunette"!

Okay, I will be the first to admit that we were both shallow and judging the girls by their appearances, their smiles, and how they carried themselves, but my point here is that we were each attracted to different girls. We each defined beauty *differently.*

Of course, when discussing attraction, it is more than physical beauty that draws and holds a man's interest in a woman.

Now, it is a scientific fact that men are, in general, more visual creatures. But even *what* we visibly notice varies from man to man. Most women believe that the first feature a man notices is how well-endowed she is, which is why breast augmentation is the number one surgical cosmetic procedure among women – with 399,440 performed in 2007. Other women pay for and endure liposuction and other expensive and painful plastic surgeries, in an attempt to conform to an idealized image of beauty and what they believe men are looking for. While, for some men, these are important attributes, the reality is that a woman's smile, self-confidence, and attitude have an even more profound effect upon how she is perceived.

Obviously, since beauty is equated with sex appeal, a physical attraction must be present, but in no way can a pretty face overcome a repulsive personality. Physical beauty may attract initial attention, but it is the inner beauty that will maintain the attraction.

First impressions always stand out in a person's mind, so it is important to take pride in your appearance, but it's equally important to project an image of your total beauty. This begins by embracing your personality and projecting your inner self-confidence. Nothing is sexier than to see a woman who feels attractive and happy with herself. Simple acts like flashing a smile or maintaining eye contact across the room not only demonstrate an interest in socializing, but also display a look of self-assurance and attractiveness that cannot be ignored.

My goal is to show you that you *are* beautiful and how to accentuate your best features – inside and out! Obviously, there's no getting around the fact that beauty not only comes from the image you project, but is also dependent upon the perception of others. As such, it is critical to understand that, since you can only control one half of that equation, happiness relies upon being content with the image of beauty you project, and not counting on gaining approval from others. The opinions, interpretations, and perceptions of beauty by others cannot be controlled, but you can learn to love yourself and control your opinion of yourself by acknowledging your beauty – and that is where real beauty starts. When you love yourself, you can't help but exude confidence. And that confidence is contagious and attention-getting.

As stated by the 19th century author Stendhal, "Beauty is no more than the promise of happiness." In order to realize this promise, you must focus on accepting yourself for who you are and striving to be the best *you* can possibly be – and take your focus off trying to attain artificially ideal standards. This means realizing, accepting, and improving upon those traits that make you a beautiful and unique individual, not despising certain other traits, all of which make you who you are. You must realize your own beauty before others will see you as beautiful. Every person in this world is an individual with a unique beauty that no other can possess – and if you constantly compare yourself to others, you're not really appreciating the beauty found in your individuality.

Self-Acceptance = Self-Confidence

Sometimes we are so concerned about what others are thinking about us. Guess what? They are doing exactly the same thing.

Imagine being able to see yourself for the beautiful person you are. Once you are able to do that, you can finally let go of the negative images you carry about yourself, opening up your mental energies to think more about others – and allowing you to build more rewarding relationships.

Picture each person that you come in contact with as having an "Emotional Bank Account." Each interaction with them either makes a positive emotional deposit into *or* a negative emotional withdrawal out of their account. Loving and focusing on others is a very attractive quality. Practice making a positive emotional deposit with each person you encounter. Give them a compliment on one of their positive attributes and watch your positive "emotional bank deposits" come back to you – with interest!

Dressing Up Inner Beauty

Stop. Look in the mirror again. List what you believe are your top three features. Now, realize that whatever you think your best features are, each person you meet may agree or disagree and may, in fact, appreciate entirely different features.

As far as men go, some prefer women with long hair, others with short hair; some prefer women that are thin, while others prefer women that are more average in weight or plus-size; some prefer women with smaller breasts, while others prefer well-endowed women; some prefer a strong-willed, driven woman, while others prefer women that are more easy-going or even submissive; some prefer women that are constantly active, while others want to meet a woman that likes to relax and just hang-out. I could go on and on, but the reality is, no matter what the personality trait or the physical feature, women can be found at both ends of the spectrum and all points in between – and there are men that appreciate the women along every part of that continuum. Let's face it, what is the first trait you notice in a person? What traits make them most attractive to you? Do you think these are the exact same traits your best friend appreciates? Do you reject any man who doesn't look like a male cover model or Hollywood star?

So, beauty is not about focusing on what you feel you are missing or what you would like to change. Beauty is a projection of confidence and contentment with what you have been given and have to offer. You do not have to change yourself to be beautiful, but you must embrace and, perhaps, accentuate and flaunt the beautiful qualities you already have. If you are constantly preoccupied with what you are missing or what you don't have, none of your time is spent projecting confidence in yourself. Since beauty is an outward projection, you can enhance the quality of those features that make you beautiful by focusing your attention on what you have instead of what you may be lacking.

There was a very old lady who loved life and had incredible self confidence. Well, over the years she had been losing her hair. One morning she went to the mirror and saw three hairs remaining. Being so positive, she said, "I think I will braid my hair today." And braid her hair she did – and continued to have a great day.

Some time later, she lost one of the hairs. She looked in the mirror and saw only two hairs remaining. "Hmmm, two hairs. Today, I think I will part my hair down the middle." And so she did, one hair to the left, the other to the right – and off she went to have a great day.

More time passed and she lost another hair. She looked in the mirror and saw the one remaining hair. "Wow, one hair! I know, a pony-tail will look just perfect!" – and off she went to have a great day.

Finally, she lost her last hair. She looked in the mirror. "How wonderful, I am finally bald. Now I won't have to waste time doing my hair anymore!" – and off she went to have a great day.

It's all about how you see yourself. **Beauty starts with confidence.**

Wasting your time agonizing over your insecurities does not allow time to be secure and pleased with yourself. If you endorse your own feelings of unattractiveness and persist in failing to find yourself beautiful, how can you truly expect others to see you as beautiful? When you focus all your attention on your imperfections, then you consciously or unconsciously broadcast your flaws to those around you, instead of the traits that make you beautiful. True beauty comes from within and from those features that make you an individual, not from meeting the requirements that define artificial ideals and stereotypes of beauty.

What most women don't understand is that when a woman feels confident in her skin, she exudes a glow that outshines anything she could wear. Let's face it, as an authority in the beauty industry, I have had the opportunity to meet all types of people - beauty editors, makeup artists, celebrities, and fashion and cover models. But no matter how "perfect" the woman was on the outside, her attitude and smile (or lack thereof) actually *redefined* her beauty.

Women need to realize that beauty does not mean conforming to look like the millions, but standing out as the uniquely beautiful one in a million! Beauty is more than appearance, it is an attitude of acceptance and happiness with yourself; it is a confidence in your talents - and it requires owning your beauty. Owning your beauty means accepting your flaws and playing up your eye-catching traits!

Olympic athletes claim that sports and endurance is 90% mental and only 10% physical talent. Similarly, beauty is 90%

inner confidence and, also, only 10% physical. Beauty manifests itself externally, but is largely comprised of the attitudes from within an individual. If discontentment or disgust with any part of oneself exists, that attitude of dissatisfaction and those feelings of unattractiveness will shine through for others to see. In addition, by revealing your own dissatisfaction with your imperfections, you make it easier for others to notice those blemishes that otherwise would likely have been overlooked, or even appreciated. Conversely, when you know yourself and are content, you are able to let go of the insecurities that consume you – allowing your playful, fun side to shine through.

When I was in high school, learning the various skills I would need to go off on my own and be an adult, I learned to cook. I would spend hours practicing. Some things definitely came out better than others, but it was fun. Well, to save myself embarrassment and to hide the insecurities I felt about my cooking, I would always say something negative when I served the meal: "I probably shouldn't have cooked it as long as I did," "I probably should have used a bit more seasoning," or "I hope you like it; It really didn't come out the way I planned."

After a while, my father got frustrated with me. And I learned a big lesson. Each meal I served, he enjoyed. He never saw the imperfections – until I pointed them out.

From that day forward, I kept my mouth shut. People have been enjoying my cooking ever since – I was even written up in the food section of our local paper once.

How many times do you make a negative comment about your own cooking? How about your makeup? Your outfit? Your weight? Have you ever asked, "Do I look fat in this?" I'll bet that no one would have noticed any imperfections - not until *you* pointed them out.

If anything, you should seek to accentuate the positive and not dwell on the negative. Real beauty is about being true to yourself and not projecting a false image to gain acceptance. But by broadcasting your own dissatisfaction with your imperfections, you make it easier for others to notice those blemishes that probably would have been overlooked or even appreciated as an attribute. It is important to remember that those who love us do not see our flaws and shortcomings, but see us as free of blemishes and flaws.

Unlike men, who focus on the qualities that make a woman beautiful, women obsess over those qualities they see as making them unattractive. I have not yet encountered a model who did not have a mole, scar, or birth mark of some sort that she despised, instead of appreciating the uniqueness it brought to her beauty. My point is that even those women that a given society considers to be the most beautiful are still seeking perfection, themselves - trained to remain insecure and find every flaw possible to fix. As an example, some of these women tan regularly to get that bronzed tone, which to them defines sex appeal - only to find years later that their leathery, sun-damaged skin makes them feel more unattractive than if they had cared for their skin without subjecting it to sun damage. Seeking perfection has consequences and is a vicious cycle.

Women must realize that beauty is an individual concept and that not all individuals define beauty the same way - and that is a good thing! *Inner* beauty comes from knowing your innermost desires and what makes you a unique individual. The gifts you contribute to the world and the attitude you project through your actions define your inner beauty. Recognizing and embracing the qualities that make you stand out from others, rather than despising your distinctive attributes, helps strengthen inner beauty. *Outer* beauty is simply a projection of the God-given physical attributes of each individual, combined with an element of personal style. Outer beauty is also an expression of personality - expressed by both the way you care for yourself and the styles you incorporate into your image. In a society fixated on externals, the amount of emphasis placed on outer beauty stops many women from taking time to reflect on the inner beauty that contributes so importantly to their total image of beauty, as perceived by others. Regardless of how beautiful you may be externally, if your personality does not match your outer beauty, then the true image of beauty you project may be significantly different than the image you perceive. In the end, congruence between outer beauty and inner beauty reflects a positively beautiful image to others.

At the end of the day, it is your inner beauty that allows you to create meaningful relationships with others and impact their lives, and it is critical to remember that this is what matters most - and what you will be remembered for in the end.

Bubble Up!

Our world is filled with images and influences. Magazines, advertisements, our favorite television shows, the news, office "water cooler" gossip – all influence us. Are you ready for a change? I mean really ready for a change? This one will make a meaningful difference, not just in how you view yourself, but in how you view others, your job, and just about every other aspect of your life.

Before you read further, I want to present a two-week "Bubble Up Challenge"! This is an easy challenge that will be fun and will truly change your life – but you must promise to try it for two weeks. If you are not truly committed to this, I mean one hundred percent committed, then jump ahead to the next chapter. But if you are serious and really want to make a positive change in your life, keep reading.

We are going to build an imaginary purple bubble around you. That's right; you now have an imaginary purple bubble around you. You are now in your own private world. The only things allowed inside are positive influences; all the negative influences are stuck on the outside.

First, stop watching the news and stop reading the newspaper. That's right. Stop. News is filled with negative stories and dramas meant to shock you, hook you in, and keep you hanging on the edge of your seat to find out if it's a major crime, some political event, a poor economy, or some other negative event that really has no bearing on your day-to-day life. I am serious. You have been conditioned to want to know all the news, but what bearing does it have on your everyday life? This step isn't about missing out on any important world events, it's about focusing on positive information and things within your sphere (or purple bubble) of control, or which have a direct impact upon your life. It's also about recognizing just how distracting - and, ultimately, meaningless or even detrimental - so many of these influences really are. Leave the news outside your bubble. Don't worry, if anything major happens, your friends will tell you.

Next, put away the fashion and celebrity magazines. These are filled with gossip passed off as news and "aspirational" images, lifestyle commentary, and advertisements to keep you wanting...and buying. For these two weeks, take a closer at your own image and your own lifestyle. And, instead of wanting more and more, focus on appreciating what you have. Believe me, the celebrity scandals and seasonal "must have" advice will still be there when the two weeks are up. But, for now, they stay outside of your bubble.

Next, stop the negative gossip. When you are at the office or around friends and they start to say something negative about someone or start complaining about something, simply say "Oh, I know her. She's one of my best friends." Even if you have never met her, it will stop the gossip in its tracks. Also, let your friends know what you are doing - and try to change the topic to something positive. This may solve the issue for you and even help them make a positive change, as well. Remember, this is not a judgment of them; they just don't know better or don't realize how harmful negative comments can be. Distance yourself from all negative influences.

Next, go out of your way to surround yourself with positive influences. Call that friend that always sees the good in every situation - yes, the one that you used to think was nuts. Maybe after you spend a few days in her world, seeing things her way, you will realize you have learned her secret to a happy, confident life. It's all about how you look at things and how you let things influence you. Friends like this we definitely want to let inside our bubble - our new world!

Finally, work on looking for the positive in every situation. Seriously. If you get a flat tire on the way home from work, what could be good about that? Maybe the delay helps you miss a traffic jam or avoid an accident. Stuck in a traffic jam? Wow, the extra time will give you a few more moments to enjoy your favorite music, call a friend on the cell phone or enjoy the company of the person riding with you. If your boss does something you don't agree with or a co-worker gets promoted, even when you know you deserve it so much more, let it go. In the meantime, you have a job. A large number of people don't - at least you are able to feed your family. You have a lot to be thankful for, and you can either enjoy each day or let things get to you and ruin your day. It is completely within your control.

I promise that, within just a few days, you are going to feel stress melt away. You will realize just how much all of these negative influences really affect us - our stress levels, our reactions to others, how we treat our children and significant others, even our health. Now that your life is quickly improving, you will start to see a smile that is genuine and from the inside. And, of course, this new confidence and positive outlook will come through for others to see. You will look and feel beautiful, emanating from the inside. Let your new purple-bubble world lift you up! Bubble up!

Try this for just two weeks and see if it doesn't make an overwhelmingly positive difference in your life! Then, let's spread the word to others and encourage them to do the same: go to my website www.JustAskDavid.com and share your Bubble-Up story with everyone! Help encourage others by sharing your story.

GIRLS' NIGHT!

There are many factors that influence our self-esteem, including the media, our family, our friends, our relationships, etc. We have already discussed how various media influences have affected our perspectives and how we feel about ourselves – and the power of eliminating negative influences.

This activity will help you and others you care about feel more confident. Ask your best friend or maybe even a few friends to come over for a girls' night! Relax. Light candles. Serve a few of your favorite foods. Go outside your comfort zone and discuss this book and how you want to try something that will change your definition of beauty and help to improve your view of yourself. Any true friend will want to help you – and herself!

1. **Pick a theme!**
   (See next page for suggestions)

2. Light pretty scented candles

3. Play mood music lightly in the background

4. Make copies or download and print copies of Girls' Night – Conversation Starters on page 27 for each guest

5. Download and print bookmarks from www.JustAskDavid.com site as Party Favors

6. Enjoy the night with friends, while discussing this book and the Conversation Starters

Suggested Themes *(on next page)*

*** Go to **www.JustAskDavid.com** and post some ideas of your own to share with everyone! ***

Babes and Books - Decorate with books stacked around the room or dessert table, play mood music, light pretty scented candles and serve desserts with herbal tea. Enjoy the evening of conversation and fun, while tasting desserts and sipping tea.

Beauty and Brains - Decorate with makeup, hair styling products, nail polish, etc. Give each other mini-makeovers. Enjoy the evening of conversation and fun, while getting a makeover.

Toes and Prose - Decorate with colorful basins you can get at any dollar store for do-it-yourself pedicures. Sprinkle glass marbles into the basins to massage toes while they soak in scented bath gel. Enjoy the evening of conversation and fun, while you soak your feet.

Coffee and Conversation - Decorate with bags of coffee or small burlap bags, coffee mugs, etc. Serve coffee and cookies. Enjoy the evening of conversation and fun, while sipping coffee and dipping cookies.

Margaritas and Meaning - Decorate with a Mexican theme, serve margaritas with chips and salsa. Enjoy the evening of conversation and fun, while sipping margaritas.

Girls' Night - Conversation Starters

The items on the next page are points for discussion. The goal is to help you realize a few things about yourself that you may never have considered. By discussing these topics with your friends, you will be able to get different points of view - and quickly realize how beautiful you really are, just as you are. Hand out the copies of the Girls' Night - Conversation Starters you made for each party guest and have each guest fill in the blanks. When you are done, you will discuss them with each other. You will soon discover that you are not alone in your insecurity - each of us has similar concerns. More importantly, you will each discover those aspects of your beauty that you may not have previously recognized, but that your friends did - and may even be jealous of. Even *more* importantly, you will all realize the power and ease with which we can help each other see the best in ourselves!

My definition of beauty is

_____

_____

People tell me I look like

_____

_____

I think I actually look like

_____

_____

I think my best traits are

_____

_____

To me, being beautiful means

_____

_____

The following traits make me unique

_____

_____

What I would most like to change about myself is

_____

_____

_____

_____

makes me feel good about myself.

_____

_____

makes me doubt myself.

Now, discuss with each other what you wrote. You will quickly learn that your perceptions are far from reality and have been tainted by the negative influences of the media and the beauty industry.

As further reinforcement, try this activity again – this time, with your newfound knowledge and perspective.

~ Chapter Two ~

Beauty From Within

Picture being on a train and going on an incredible journey from point A to point B. The ride is so much fun you just don't want it to end. Reality is, that train is going to get there – but if you could only slow down that train and extend the ride! Now imagine that journey is your life. What would you do to extend the ride and increase the enjoyment of it? To be healthy and in the best shape possible? To look and feel your best for that ride?

One of my friends pointed out to me, "It's not the years in your life, but the life into those years that matters most." Obviously, my friend was talking about the *quality* of life, which is made up of many things. Most often when discussing quality of life, we talk about the experiences we pack into it, but it is also important to discuss your ability to enjoy those experiences, which depends, in large part, upon your health. More than any other factor, what you eat affects your body – and your skin. Understanding this is very important if you want to stay as healthy and youthful as possible – and make the most out of every minute!

Relax. This isn't another book telling you to diet and what you can or cannot eat. You are an adult. You are capable of making your own decisions – as long as you have the facts. My goal is to give you those facts. In this chapter, you will learn about some of the key factors that play a role in beautiful skin, as well as suggestions for foods you can incorporate into your diet that can have a significant influence. I talk about skin for two reasons. First, because this is a book about beauty and looking your best starts with creating and maintaining healthy skin. The second reason is because the health and appearance of your skin can often tell you a lot about your internal health.

Being beautiful goes beyond healthy skin and includes having a healthy body. What you put into your body, including food and nutritional supplements, affects how you feel and how you look, including the firmness and youthfulness of your skin. This chapter is your recipe for "internal skin care."

What's On Tap?

Let's start with the most critical part of our diet – water. Our bodies are comprised of about 70% water. It is essential to keep our bodies well hydrated and, in turn, our skin cells hydrated – from the inside out. Typically, we lose about 2 to 2.5 liters of water each day through perspiration, breathing, and our other normal bodily functions. We need to replace that fluid every day. Our food intake replaces about 20% of the fluids, while the remaining amount comes from consumption of beverages. Following the common "8x8" rule of drinking eight 8-ounce glasses of liquid provides 64 ounces or approximately 1.9 liters. While you can consume a variety of beverages to achieve this goal, pure, clean water provides the greatest benefit.

What kind of water do you drink? I know what you are thinking – "What type of water?" But it really does make a difference. Water is not just water. While all this sounds like double talk and you might think you are doing your body well by drinking glass after glass of water every day, evidence shows that plain old tap water contains elements that can be detrimental to your skin – even accelerate the signs of aging.

Plain tap water, which millions of Americans drink every day, can contain over 300 contaminants. While there are regulations on some of the chemicals found in our water supply, more than half of the chemicals can legally be present – *at any level* – and are not subject to any governmental regulations. While I could write a separate book just on water and contaminants, I will focus on tap water and how it affects your skin.

Tap water contains:

- HEAVY METALS – such as lead, iron, copper, magnesium, calcium and zinc
- SALTS & MINERALS – contaminants that can actually cause skin dryness
- CHEMICALS – such as fluoride and chlorine, which are added by our own water treatment plants

Every time you take a drink, you are exposing your body to these contaminants. Every time you take a bath, shower, or even wash your face, you are exposing your skin to these contaminants. Your water is attacking you and your skin from the outside *and* the inside.

What kind of damage can result?

WRINKLES: Heavy metals can oxidize and create a chain reaction that generates free radicals. These free radicals attack and destroy collagen fibers. The loss of collagen results in the appearance of fine lines, crow's feet, and deep wrinkles.

ACNE & ENLARGED PORES: Heavy metals convert the skin's natural oils into a hard, waxy type of substance that clogs pores, leading to blackheads, whiteheads, pimples, and enlarged pores.

ECZEMA, REDNESS & SKIN STRESS: Heavy metals and other impurities can irritate the skin, creating skin stress, redness, and promoting the symptoms of eczema.

What Can You Do?

FORGET BOTTLED WATER: So, what should you drink? Forget bottled water! Do yourself a favor - go read the label on your favorite bottled water. Read it carefully. While pictures of mountains lead most consumers to imagine the water is clean, natural spring water, you may now have discovered words similar to "purified water" or "bottled from municipal sources" on the label, which means it is simply filtered tap water. This is common practice for many companies, including some of the largest and most popular brands. But, despite the labeling, you still won't know if the water is processed, polluted, packaged tap water. The Environmental Working Group (EWG) found 38 contaminants in 10 popular brands.

> Each year, we consume and dispose of an estimated 30 BILLION plastic water bottles. While 80% of the U.S. households have access to plastic recycling programs, it is reported that only 23% of PET bottles are actually recycled. That means almost 80% of every plastic water bottle ends up in our landfills.

FILTERED WATER: Contact Culligan, visit your local Home Depot, Lowe's®, or other discount retailer and find a certified water filtration system. There are many options available, at a range of costs and a variety of filtration levels. My favorite is a reverse osmosis system, which is a little costlier - but extremely effective. If possible, install one for the entire house. If not, get one for your kitchen sink and even consider one for your ice maker. The filtered water should be your source for everything from cooking to quenching your thirst to making ice. Then consider a filter for the shower for bathing - showerhead filters are readily available. Remember, we are looking at everything that affects you inside and out!

Picking the Right Foods

Incorporating the right foods into your diet is essential for optimum health and beauty. All foods contain an array of proteins, nutrients, micro-nutrients, and chemical compounds - eating the right kinds of food provides the building blocks for healthy cell regeneration. Eating a variety of different healthy foods will help ensure you are giving your body what it needs to keep you beautiful.

EFAs = Essentials For Ageless Skin

Our bodies need a range fatty acids for biological processes that regulate and affect a wide range of functions, including blood pressure, blood clotting, inflammation, immunity, joint function, skin health, hair growth, and so much more. EFAs can also dilute sebum, helping to prevent pores from clogging (and problems with acne). Our bodies can produce all the fatty acids they need, except for two: Alpha-Linolenic Acid and Linoleic Acid – both of which are unsaturated fats, more commonly known as Omega-3 and Omega-6.

These two fatty acids are also known as Essential Fatty Acids. While Essential Fatty Acids are necessary for proper health, the body cannot produce them. EFAs must be taken internally through diet or nutritional supplements. Most people probably already get enough Omega-6 from the foods they eat, but many people are deficient in their consumption of Omega-3.

WHAT TO EAT: Eat foods rich in Omega-3 and Omega-6 two or three times each week, such as cold-water fish – salmon, halibut, and tuna. Plus, incorporate extra virgin olive oil, wheat germ oil, and cold-pressed flaxseed oil in your salads for an extra one to two tablespoons each day. A good snack includes raw pumpkin seeds. If you are not a big fish eater, you may want to consider Omega-3 and Omega-6 nutritional supplements.

Collagen Building Blocks

Collagen is a group of naturally-occurring proteins and accounts for approximately 75% of our skin tissue. Collagen's key role is to provide strength, elasticity and support to the skin.

However, starting at the young age of 25, our Collagen levels begin to deplete at the rate of 1.5% each year. By the time a woman reaches menopause, a whopping forty-five percent of Collagen is lost. The loss of Collagen leads to loss of firmness, leading to the appearance of wrinkles.

Collagen cannot be absorbed topically into the skin, so the key is to topically use ingredients that will promote Collagen synthesis (discussed more later on) and to include key Collagen-promoting foods into our diets. Remember, Collagen is comprised of protein, so a protein-rich diet is critical.

WHAT TO EAT: I am not a fan of powdered Collagen. Consider adjusting your diet to include foods that will work with the body's natural processes. For breakfast, include eggs a few times a week. If you are worried about cholesterol, egg whites will do the trick! For lunch and dinner, include meats like chicken, fish, and beef (preferably lean). Low-fat yogurt, cottage cheese, nuts, and seeds are all good too.

Vitamin C is not only essential for building Collagen, it is also a powerful anti-oxidant. Make sure your daily intake includes fruit and fruit juices from oranges, grapefruits, papayas, strawberries and kiwis. As side dishes with your meals, include vegetables that are high in Vitamin C, such as tomatoes, cauliflower, broccoli, red peppers and Brussels sprouts.

Hyaluronic Acid
- Miracle Moisturizer & Essential Anti-Aging Element

Another building block is Hyaluronic Acid, a member of the glycosaminoglycan family, which is found within collagen in every tissue of our body, with the highest concentrations occurring in our connective tissues, such as skin and cartilage. Hyaluronic Acid forms a viscous fluid with exceptional lubricating properties. This is necessary for the vital functions of many parts of the human body, including the skin, heart valves, aqueous/vitreous portion of the eye, and synovial fluid (joint cushion and lubricant). Hyaluronic Acid acts as a water magnet, holding more water than any other molecule in the body, and is necessary to the structure of connective tissue and for keeping collagen hydrated and tissue youthful. Considering that our bodies metabolize or excrete as much as 100-150mg of Hyaluronic Acid each day, it makes sense to include it in our daily nutritional supplement plan and topical skin care program – especially for those over the age of 50.

WHAT TO EAT: Salads are important. Tomatoes and leafy green vegetables, such as spinach and kale, are reported to be high in Hyaluronic Acid. While root vegetables, like potatoes and sweet potatoes, are also a good source, Hyaluronic Acid is sensitive to heat and is destroyed by cooking the vegetables. Additionally, drink plenty of water. The effectiveness of Hyaluronic Acid is dramatically improved when you are well-hydrated and there is plenty of water to bind to.

Super Anti-Oxidants, Super Fruits

Free radicals are the ultimate enemy and can damage the skin. Free radicals are unstable oxygen molecules with an unpaired number of electrons. In an effort to stabilize themselves, these highly reactive molecules try to "rip away" an electron from a healthy cell, thereby damaging the healthy cell. The end result is a chain reaction that is one of the reasons our organs and tissues age. What causes free radicals? Well, free radicals form naturally in the body; however, the process is accelerated by smoking, pollution, sunlight exposure, high-fat and high-sugar diets, and excessive amounts of alcohol.

WHAT TO EAT: Antioxidants are molecules that interact with and neutralize these free radicals – before vital cells are damaged. Essentially, they safely "lend" an electron to the unstable oxygen molecule. There are a number of fruits, vegetables, and even certain spices that are high in antioxidants. The National Institute on Aging developed a method of measuring the antioxidant capacity of different foods and nutritional supplements called ORAC (Oxygen Radical Absorbance Capacity) value.

Blueberries, pomegranates, kiwi fruit, broccoli, spinach, tomatoes, soy, oats, and even dark chocolate have high ORAC values and offer significant antioxidant properties. Or, consider various nutritional supplements that contain CoQ10, Vitamin A, Vitamin C, Vitamin E, Beta-Carotene, Lycopene, Ginkgo Biloba, and Grape Seed Extract.

For a more complete list, visit www.JustAskDavid.com in Resources – ORAC Values.

SUPPLEMENTS

Resveratrol: America's #1 Anti-Aging Molecule

For almost twenty years, scientists have studied why some cultures that enjoy red wine on a regular basis have fewer health problems. Some call it the "French paradox." The answer they found lies in a substance called Resveratrol – a polyphenol naturally derived from the skin of red wine grapes, certain berries, and certain other plants.

Scientific studies have shown that Resveratrol, especially when combined with other polyphenols, has significant anti-aging effects, providing superior anti-oxidant protection, as well as supporting a healthy lifestyle and anti-inflammatory response.

Let's be clear, Resveratrol isn't going to magically turn a 70-year-old into a 20-year-old. However, in testing, Resveratrol has demonstrated properties that provide a major breakthrough in the war against the signs of aging.

Resveratrol has been such a ground-breaking discovery in anti-aging research, it has been featured on CNN, 60 Minutes, Barbara Walters, Fox News, Web MD, and numerous news programs.

WHAT TO EAT: While there are Resveratrol capsules on the market, the key is finding the right source with the highest level possible. One suggestion is a liquid concentrate of Resveratrol - polyphenols derived from the skin of red wine grapes, combined with Organic Acai Berry, Goji Berry, Pomegranate, and a combination of other nutrient-rich berries. There are a number of potentially effective supplements on the market. One that I have found and like provides a proprietary blend that delivers the daily Resveratrol benefits equivalent to 3,000 glasses of red wine. Check out my website **www.JustAskDavid.com** and try it!

Vitamins

A multi-vitamin is not the cure for a poor diet. However, if you're eating right, boosting your diet with specific foods and nutritional supplements can make a difference.

There are two types of vitamins:

1. Water Soluble Vitamins

2. Fat Soluble Vitamins

WATER SOLUBLE

Water soluble vitamins, such as B-Complex Vitamins and Vitamin C, dissolve quickly in water. As such, these vitamins cannot be stored by your body and must be a part of your daily diet.

FAT SOLUBLE

Since these vitamins are soluble in fat, excess amounts can be stored by the body for days or even months. Fat soluble Vitamins include A, D, E and K

Vitamin A promotes proper cell function and is reported to help reduce the amount of sebum produced, which is why Vitamin A is often used by doctors in the treatment of acne. While Vitamin A has its benefits, it has concerns as well (including taking too much) – but more from a topical use, which is discussed later in this book.

Vitamin B3, also known as Niacin, helps detoxify the body and promotes proper metabolizing of protein and fat.

Vitamin C is a powerful antioxidant, is essential for tissue growth, promotes collagen synthesis, and helps in wound healing.

Vitamin D promotes cell growth and helps repair damage to the skin's structure.

Vitamin E is an anti-inflammatory, as well as providing antioxidant benefits to help protect cell membranes.

Vitamin K helps strengthen bones and capillaries. However, taking more than the recommended amounts of Vitamin K can cause liver damage or problems for those taking blood-thinning drugs. See your doctor before taking any supplements with Vitamin K.

What Not To Eat

Just as improving what you eat can provide tremendous benefits for looking and feeling younger, eating the wrong foods can counteract your efforts. Obviously, foods that contribute to fat gain can impact your overall appearance, but, more specifically, consuming certain foods in excess can have a negative effect on your skin – and accelerate the visible signs of aging:

High Salt Content foods can contribute to drier skin, cause puffiness, especially around the eyes, aggravate skin redness, and even contribute to breakouts. These types of foods include sandwich meats, frozen dinners, canned foods, and several types of snack foods, including chips, crackers, and pretzels. Read the nutritional labels to determine sodium (salt) content.

Fried Foods & Snacks are high in saturated and, often, trans fats that can clog pores and promote breakouts.

Refined Carbohydrates can cause a spike in blood sugar and harm the skin in the long run. These foods include pasta, white rice, breads, and other white flour products; also, those made with refined sweeteners, like white sugar, corn syrup, and high-fructose corn syrup. Sugar, in excess, can damage collagen and elastin, resulting in an increase in lines and wrinkles. Alcohol dilates blood vessels in the skin, increases skin redness, aggravates rosacea, and causes a flushed appearance.

Putting Life In Your Years

I will admit that I am addicted to my morning coffee. So, please understand, this is not about stopping everything you enjoy. Rather, I wanted to provide you with a little of the basic information you need to evaluate some of the things you currently eat and drink and give you "food for thought" (I know, forgive the pun) on how you can improve your overall eating habits for improved cellular health, which will help you look and feel younger for the long term. If this section has struck a chord with you, I would encourage you to do more research.

Remember, the train is going from point A to point B. We want to extend that ride and enjoy every possible moment by being in our best possible shape for that ride.

~ Chapter Three ~

The Truth About What's Inside

The Truth About What's Inside

If you have ever traveled a lot, you know how difficult it is to be away from your family – just like the guy in this story that I want to share with you. Well, a "road warrior" was used to taking short one- and two-day trips. This time, he had to travel for almost two weeks. Traveling home, his flight was delayed and then hit rough weather the entire flight back. Throughout the entire flight, he kept picturing how nice it was going to be to get home and be able to lay next to his wife and just hold her – and his little kids who would be so excited to see him at breakfast the next morning.

The flight landed in the storm. It was very late. He drove-his car home. The entire drive it was pouring rain, thunder crashing. He finally arrived home to find his kids in bed with their mom. So, not wanting to wake anyone, he slept on the couch.

The next morning, everyone was so happy to see each other. Even so, the dad decided to explain to the kids, "When I am away, I miss each of you so much. I look forward to coming home to see mommy and you kids. Now, I understand if you are so scared that you want to sleep in our room, but the nights I come home, it would be nice if you slept in your own rooms." The kids told their dad, "no problem!"

Well a few months went by with more short trips; finally, the dad was faced with another two-week trip. Again, during the entire flight home he pictured being able to see his family. This time, he landed on a Saturday afternoon, so the family planned to meet him at the airport. He couldn't wait. The flight landed. He gathered his things, walked down the jet-way, through the terminal, and exited security to see his family waiting among the crowd.

His youngest raced out all excited, proud to share some news, and yelled out loudly, "Daddy! Daddy! Guess What? This time you were away, nobody slept with mommy!"

Every head in the terminal turned toward him and a dead silence fell over everyone in the terminal. The dad turned red and didn't know what to say. He understood what his son meant – and wanted to explain to each and every person what his son meant – but knew that was impossible.

I guess that is how I feel right now – embarrassed and at a bit of a loss for words to explain my "family," in this case, the cosmetics industry. The cosmetics industry makes a lot of claims in advertisements, on packaging, even on ingredient statements. But there is a lot more to the story, and I want to explain it to each and every one of you!

This isn't going to make me very popular in the cosmetics industry, but I want to share with you:

- **How the Food & Drug Administration (FDA) Categorizes Personal Care Products** – you may be surprised to learn that some of the items you use every day are considered drugs
- **What Product Claims Are Really Saying**

- "Tricks of the Trade" when promoting specific ingredients
- How to Read an Ingredient Statement and determine what is really inside the products you use every day
- The Differences Between Discount Brands And Expensive Brands

How the FDA Categorizes Personal Care Products

Is It A Drug, Cosmetic, or Soap?

The FDA – or U.S. Food and Drug Administration – is the federal agency responsible for regulating all products that we put into or onto our bodies, excluding meat and poultry. This includes prescription and non-prescription drugs, vaccines, medical devices, radiological products (including cellular phones), animal drugs and feed, plus cosmetics.

For our purposes, we are going to focus on cosmetics. The definition of cosmetics is a broad term and includes much more than color cosmetics and makeup. The term cosmetics includes all personal care products and all face and body products that are not ingested – including moisturizers, serums, face cleansers, body washes, self-tanners, tanning oils, sunscreens, lipstick, eye shadow, nail polish, shampoo, hair color, permanent waves, relaxers, deodorants, anti-perspirants, and even toothpaste! Yep, even toothpaste, since it is intended to clean part of the body and not be ingested.

The FDA divides these products into two different categories...well, actually three: Drugs, Cosmetics, and Soaps. Most people think it's a particular ingredient or combination of ingredients that determines which category a given product falls into. Actually, it's the intended use of these products that determines if they are classified as a drug, cosmetic, or soap. Well, isn't it obvious? Nope.

A product is defined as a drug if it is either "intended for use in the diagnosis, cure, mitigation, treatment, or prevention of disease" or "intended to affect the structure or any function of the body." What does all that mean? The quickest and easiest way to put it is this: if the product claims to affect or change the body in any way, then it's a drug. The drug category has two sub-categories: Over-The-Counter (OTC), which does not require a prescription (non-prescription drug), and Prescription Drugs, which require a prescription. All other non-drug products would be classified as cosmetics.

So ask yourself... *Can* a cosmetic become a Drug?

Can a Cosmetic Become a Drug?

What's the difference between anti-perspirant and deodorant? Wait – before you answer, let me make it a little more difficult. What if I was in the lab, made a batch of a formulation, poured half into one roll-on container and labeled it anti-perspirant, then poured the other half into another roll-on container and labeled it deodorant? Now, what is the difference?

Careful.... Don't worry, I have yet to meet someone outside the cosmetic field that can answer the question correctly. The difference is the anti-perspirant is a drug (OTC Drug). It claims to stop perspiration, which is a physiological change or change to the function of the body. The other is a deodorant and is considered a cosmetic, since it simply claims to deodorize or cover up odor. It's neither the ingredients nor the formulation that make the difference, but rather the claims made about the product. Other examples of common products that are thought of as cosmetics, but which actually fall into the category of drugs, include anti-dandruff shampoo (since it treats a skin disorder), toothpaste with fluoride (since it prevents cavities), moisturizers with sun protection claims, etc.

Oh yeah, what about the third category: soap? Um, this one should be obvious, shouldn't it? If it walks like a duck and quacks like a duck, then it's a duck, right? Guess again. According to the FDA, if the product's detergent properties are from an *alkali salt of fatty acid* compound AND it is labeled solely as soap, then it is soap. What does that mean? Well, for a soap to be qualified as soap, it must go through a process where the core ingredients are processed with lye or some other alkali solution (extremely high pH – we'll talk more about pH and soaps later). Most common bars of soap fall into this category.

What about liquid cleansers, body washes, liquid face cleansers and shampoos? These are good examples of cleansing products that most of us would naturally consider soap, but which are technically NOT soap. Why? Because, if a product is marketed as a body cleanser that also moisturizes or beautifies, then it is a cosmetic, not a soap - which is the case with most of these types of products. There are also times where a company could label a product as soap, if they desired, but it would actually fall into the category of cosmetics for regulatory purposes.

What does all this mean? Well, it's important for you to understand the differences in how the FDA categorizes products, because the production and labeling requirements for each category vary. Non-prescription drugs and Over-the-Counter (OTC) products, such as anti-perspirants, SPF sunscreens, first aid products, cortisone creams, acne products, fluoride toothpastes, etc., have very strict requirements for labeling and manufacturing. Cosmetics, including skin creams, makeup, body lotions, self tanners, etc., do not face the same requirements. The cosmetics industry is self-regulated, meaning it's up to each manufacturer to determine standards and produce quality products that deliver what they claim. SURPRISE: The burden also falls on you, the consumer, to know how to read and understand these claims and evaluate what is inside the product. You've heard the Latin phrase, "Caveat emptor"? Literally, "Let the Buyer Beware."

Don't worry, I'm going to guide you through this process and help you to better understand the products you use currently – and help you know which products to purchase in the future.

What About Cosmeceuticals?

"Cosmeceutical" is actually just a marketing term that merges the word "cosmetic" with "pharmaceutical," hoping to imply that a product is stronger, more effective, or has some special clinical benefit. However, it is misleading. The FDA does not recognize cosmeceuticals as a category and, as such, does not have any additional requirements for products to be marketed this way. Cosmeceuticals are simply cosmetic products with a clever marketing name attached to them, allowing cosmetic companies to raise the prices on these products.

What Product Claims Are Really Saying

If that wasn't confusing enough, cosmetic companies make things even more difficult by pushing the limits of truth with product claims. Cosmetic companies understand the desires women have to look younger, look and feel better, achieve fast results, etc. So, many cosmetic claims are designed to lead your brain down a specific path. Carefully chosen words are used so that you, the consumer, read the product label and imagine it says what you want it to say.

Example of some anti-wrinkle product claims:

- "Skin Feels Firmer"
- "Overall Appearance Is Firmer And More Youthful Looking"
- "Fine Lines And Wrinkles Are Visibly Reduced"
- "Felt An Improvement In The Elasticity Of Their Skin"
- "Skin Tone, Clarity, And Texture Visibly Improved"
- "Skin Looks More Radiant And Luminous Than Before"

Now, let's review each one again, slowly. The words below that are italicized and underlined are what are known as "disclaimers." They help to keep the claim from making a statement of physiological change, and turn it, instead, into one of emotion – or one that is open to interpretation. For example, "Skin _Feels_ Firmer." Most would think that the cream is claiming to firm the skin; however, that would be a physiological change, requiring the company to qualify the product as a drug. In reality, the claim merely says how your skin will feel. It's a fine, and intentionally deceptive, line. Re-read each one again, keeping this in mind.

- Skin *Feels* Firmer
- Overall *Appearance* Is Firmer And More Youthful *Looking*
- Fine Lines And Wrinkles Are *Visibly* Reduced
- *Felt* An Improvement In The Elasticity Of Their Skin
- Skin Tone, Clarity, And Texture *Visibly* Improved
- Skin *Looks* More Radiant And Luminous Than Before

What about other types of claims like:

- "Clinically Proven"
- "Dermatologist Tested"

Tricks of the Trade

"Clinically Proven"

What does "Clinically Proven" mean? This term is another claim that is thrown around loosely. To help cosmetic companies stay on the cutting edge and introduce new products, chemical companies continuously introduce new key ingredients. To help their ingredients stand out, the chemical companies often make strong claims and perform some level of clinical testing on the raw material or ingredient.

Cosmetic companies that use the ingredient can then make the claim "Clinically Proven To..." or "Clinically Proven Technology" on their final products. This type of statement or claim can be misleading, for the following reasons:

1. **SMALL TEST GROUPS**: The raw material is often tested only on a very small group of test subjects. Since the tests are for a cosmetic product and not a drug, this is allowed. NOTE: Drug testing has a completely different level of requirements.

2. **UNKNOWN LEVELS**: During the clinical testing, a chemical manufacturer will perform the tests on a base product with a specific level or amount of the ingredient in it. However, there is no requirement for cosmetic manufacturers to use that specific level in their final products. A cosmetic manufacturer *may* use the test level, but they can also use only trace levels – and still make the claim "Clinically Proven," since the claim refers to the ingredient that was, indeed, tested and which demonstrated results.

3. RAW MATERIAL vs. FINISHED PRODUCT:

Since the testing is performed on a specific chemical, it may or may not deliver the same results when put into the finished product. Some chemicals react with each other. Some chemical interactions can enhance the delivery or performance, while others can cause harm or interfere with the performance.

** Some retailers have caught on to this practice and want the manufacturers to be more forthcoming with the end user – you! These retailers will require the cosmetic company to test the finished product to substantiate the claim; they may also require a larger test subject base. If a manufacturer is unwilling, the retailer may not allow the manufacturer to make that claim, or the retailer may decide not to carry the product at all. I intentionally did not list the retailers here, since some retailers change their requirements from time to time. You can either check my website *www.JustAskDavid.com* for the latest listings or contact the retailer's headquarters and ask what their requirements are for cosmetic testing.

I can tell you right now that a number of brands will not want to test the finished product. They will claim it is too costly. However, the real reason is that they don't know if their product will really deliver what they promise. If the manufacturer truly believes in their product's performance and wants to make sure their product delivers what they promise, the testing should really not be an issue. And while there is a cost involved, it is far less than the cost of a one-page ad in any one of the major fashion magazines.

THINGS YOU CAN DO: Write a letter to the headquarters of your favorite retailer and ask them their policy. Write to your favorite manufacturer and ask them the same question. Even suggest that they adapt their policy and then register their store or brand at www.JustAskDavid.com. You can even copy this page and send it to the retailer – after all, some retail buyers do not know the inside scoop on the "Clinically Proven" claim. They may be interested to find out.

"Dermatologist Tested"

What does it mean to you? Stop for a minute and think about it. Okay, now I'll tell you what it really means. If a product is subjected to a Repeat Insult Patch Test (RIPT) to determine the irritation and/or allergic sensitization potential, the product can then claim "Dermatologist Tested" or "Dermatologist Approved." Typically, this test is performed on fifty test subjects, where the product is placed under a patch that is worn by the test subject, who is then evaluated for irritation. This test can be from a few weeks to as many as eight weeks. While the results will help determine if a product causes irritation, the statement "Dermatologist Tested" often gives the consumer a different perception of a product – for instance, that it is *recommended* by dermatologists – especially if stated after a few dramatic claims.

"Contains X%"

Another type of claim is the listing of a percentage of a particular ingredient used in the product. Manufacturers hope that by listing the percentage of an ingredient, it will indicate a higher dosage and help set them apart from the competition. However, the percentages listed can be misleading. It's another "Trick of the Trade."

Consider the claim carefully. Some examples include:

- 10% Glycolic Acid
- 5% Vitamin K
- 99.9% Aloe Vera

Okay, so how much of each ingredient is really in the product? Don't worry, I do a lot of public speaking and educational seminars. During my talks, I ask this same question – and have never had anyone get it right, even members of the cosmetic industry. So, let's look at each claim again:

10% Glycolic Acid
Cosmetic grade Glycolic Acid is 70% active. In this example, 10% of a 70% active material translates to a true 7% of Glycolic Acid in the product. In this case, the percentage represented the volume of the finished product

that was Glycolic Acid, but because the formulation of the Glycolic Acid used was diluted, the true volume of active ingredient is actually less.

5% Vitamin K

Have you ever seen or maybe even purchased a Varicose Vein product with 5% Vitamin K? Cosmetic grade Vitamin K is available in 2% and 5% activity levels. Assume the manufacturer purchased the 5% Vitamin K material. Then, next time the manufacturing department is batching a large run of the product, they climb up the stairs to the top of the mixing tank while carrying the little bottle of 5% active Vitamin K. They open the top of the tank and sprinkle in a drop or two. Now, you just saw it - a drop or two went in - so guess what? Now the manufacturer can claim this product contains 5% Vitamin K. In this case, the 5% didn't refer to the volume of Vitamin K in the product, at all - just the concentration of the Vitamin K used, and an indication that there was even the tiniest of amounts in the finished product.

99.9% Aloe Vera

Have you ever had sunburn? Have you ever purchased an Aloe Gel with 99.9% Aloe? So, how much Aloe is really in the product? You guessed it! Aloe is available at a variety of active levels and even as a powder, which somehow allows a claim of 200% Aloe Vera. Anyway, by simply putting a drop of a 99.9% Aloe Vera solution into the gel, a claim can be made that the product "Contains 99.9% Aloe." Read the ingredients on the back of the bottle. Look for an ingredient called "Carbomer." This is a gelling agent – and is what creates the sensation of a true Aloe Vera gel, such as you would expect to get out of an actual Aloe Vera leaf.

SPF Sunscreen

There is no question that over exposure to the sun can cause skin cancer. However, recent studies show that sunscreens can help prevent sunburn, but can only help protect against one of three types of skin cancer. I think the most alarming fact is that sunscreens do not protect against melanoma - the deadliest form of skin cancer.

Of course, you should avoid the sun whenever possible. However, if not, the best forms of sun protection are the shade and protective clothing. Sunscreens are a recommended layer of protection, but not the solution.

Using sunscreens has some negative effects as well:

1. FALSE SENSE OF SECURITY:

    Some dermatologists are concerned that products labeled with high SPF ratings let people feel invincible, encouraging people to increase the time they are exposed to the sun – and, in turn, escalating the risk of skin cancer.

2. MISLEADING HIGHER SPF RATINGS:

    The FDA says that the higher SPF ratings are inherently misleading" and "...there is no assurance that the specific values themselves are in fact truthful." However, there are no regulations preventing manufacturers from making the higher SPF claims in the United States, while several countries have already issued restrictions limiting the distribution of sunscreen.

3. VITAMIN A:

    Retinol and Retinyl Palmitate are forms of Vitamin A commonly used to help fight the signs of aging. However, recent studies have shown that the use of Vitamin A in sunscreens may actually accelerate the development of skin tumors and lesions. Currently, over 40% of the sunscreens on the market today contain Retinol or Retinyl Palmitate – it is important for you to read the ingredient statement, before you make your next sunscreen purchase.

SPF Sunscreens are important to provide a layer of protection, but they are not the complete solution. Additionally, don't let the labeling mislead you. Understand the label and read the ingredient statement carefully – before making a purchase.

"Preservative Free"

To help a product sound more natural, some cosmetic companies make a claim that their product *doesn't* contain a particular ingredient. For example, some companies will claim "Preservative Free." Are these products really preservative free? Any product that is expected to last more than a few days requires a preservative. Some companies claim that the packaging is airless, allowing the company to eliminate the preservative. However, a number of these products incorporate essential oils, glycols or other ingredients that can be claimed for other purposes, while providing preservative benefits. Keep in mind, every product should have a preservative – whether natural or synthetic. So, how can a manufacturer make the claim "Preservative Free"? Any product is made of several ingredients. Each of the raw materials must be stable and able to be stored in a warehouse for a period of time. The ingredients required to make or preserve the raw material are considered insignificant and, according to the FDA, are not required to be listed on the ingredient statement. Some companies may specifically source botanical extracts or other raw materials with high levels of preservatives. By using those specific materials, the manufacturer does not need to add extra preservatives to the final product and, in turn, can state "Preservative Free." Remember, they did not add any to the final formulation. Acceptable from a regulatory standpoint? Yes. Ethical? No. Of course, not all manufacturers take advantage of these loopholes. I just want you to be aware of some very common practices in the industry, to empower you to find out about the products you use. Don't hesitate. The most important dollar any manufacturer can receive is **your dollar!** So, don't be shy, don't hesitate – ask the manufacturer of your favorite brands about any claims or ingredients you want to know more about.

Does The FDA Approve Cosmetic Products?

No. The FDA does not. The cosmetic industry is a self-regulated industry. It is the manufacturer's responsibility to ensure that products are manufactured and labeled correctly. Failure to do so may result in a product being considered misbranded, which then is subject to FDA involvement.

Additionally, the FDA does not approve cosmetic products. Thus, no cosmetic product can be labeled "FDA Approved," and any such claim is considered misbranding. However, cosmetics can be voluntarily registered with the FDA and *that* may be stated on a product or brochure. Just be aware that being registered with the FDA does not mean that the product or its claims have been evaluated or approved.

How Do I Know What's Really Inside My Products?

The ingredient statement can tell you more than you think! Based upon the category a product falls into, the rules for labeling or listing of ingredients varies. A product that falls into the drug category has strict guidelines as to what claims can be made and how the ingredients must be listed. For these, the "actives," or active ingredients, are listed with the percentage used in the product, with the remaining ingredients listed as Inactive Ingredients and listed in either descending order or alphabetical order, depending upon the type of product. When ingredients are listed in alphabetical order, the percentages of those ingredients are totally unknown.

Cosmetic products list ingredients in descending order – starting with the ingredient that represents the highest percentage of the total volume. However, there is an exception to this rule. This rule only applies to those ingredients that represent greater than 1% of the total. Ingredients used in a formulation at 1% or less can be listed in any order. In other words, a manufacturer can shuffle the list of all those ingredients used at 1% or less.

Why would a manufacturer want to do this? Simple. Remember the Vitamin K in our earlier example? They do this to make it appear that there is a higher amount of certain ingredients that consumers are looking for, or maybe to imply a lesser amount of undesirable ingredients that manufacturers want to downplay.

So how do you know what's really in your skin care?

1. Make a photocopy of the ingredient statement or print it out from an online retailer's website.

2. Highlight the section of ingredients that are typically used at 1% or less. Some of the most common ingredients that are rarely, if ever, used above 1% include:

    - Vitamins and Vitamin Derivatives, often listed as Retinyl Palmitate (Vitamin A), Retinol (Vitamin A), Tocopherol Acetate (Vitamin E), Ubiquinone (CoQ10)
    - Thickeners, such as Carbomer, Xanthan Gum, Hydroxyethylcellulose, Magnesium Aluminum Silicate, or other types of Cellulose
    - Fragrance, which would typically also include essential oils
    - Colorants (if any)
    - Preservatives, which include Methylparaben, Propylparaben, Phenoxyehtanol, Methylisothiazolinone, Dehydroacetic Acid, Benzyl Alcohol, Potassium Sorbate
    - Others, such as Polysorbate, Acrylates Copolymer, Dimethicone, Triethanolamine, Aminomethyl Propanol, TEA, EDTA, BHT, BHA

3. Review the ingredient statement and see if the key ingredients being touted are listed before the area you have just highlighted. If so, the ingredient is most likely used at a level above 1%. If the ingredient comes after any of the ingredients you have just highlighted, the ingredient in question was most likely not used at a level above 1% and may, therefore, be listed in misleading order.

"Fairy Dusting" and "Magic Dust" are terms often used by manufacturers, referring to the listing of ingredients perceived by consumers to be important or highly effective – yet which are only sprinkled into the batch at trace levels. Is this legal? Yes, any ingredient that goes into the product – even at trace levels – gets listed. Remember, the "Magic Dust" ingredients can appear in any order within the group of ingredients at 1% or less. That is why I think it's important for EVERYONE to know how to read an ingredient statement and understand where the 1% level really begins – and realize that from that point all the way through the rest of the ingredient statement, any active ingredient listed is present at a low level.

Practice Your New Skills For Understanding

Ingredient Statements

Here is a sample ingredient statement for a product that makes the following claims and retails for $45 per half ounce (that's $90 per ounce):

- "Seven natural ingredients to target under eye circles"
- "Reduce puffiness"
- "Restore moisture"

Take a moment and highlight the ingredients that are typically at 1% or less.

Water, Propylene Glycol, Polyacrylamide, C13 14 Isoparaffin, Phenoxyethanol, Methylparaben, Sodium Metabisulfite, Laureth 7, Sodium Ascorbyl Phosphate, Disodium EDTA, Sodium PCA, Propylparaben, Sodium Hyaluronate, Chamomilla Recutita Flower Oil (Matricaria), Camellia Sinensis Leaf Extract, Vanillin

Now, compare your highlighted list with the one I have highlighted below. Did you catch these?

> Water, Propylene Glycol, Polyacrylamide, C13 14 Isoparaffin, Phenoxyethanol, Methylparaben, Sodium Metabisulfite, Laureth 7, Sodium Ascorbyl Phosphate, Disodium EDTA, Sodium PCA, Propylparaben, Sodium Hyaluronate, Chamomilla Recutita Flower Oil (Matricaria), Camellia Sinensis Leaf Extract, Vanillin

If only the first four ingredients are at 1% or above, does the remaining combination of ingredients really warrant $45 per half ounce? What can the level of the seven natural ingredients claimed to deliver the promised results truly be? Is it likely you're getting your money's worth?

Do Cosmetics Have Expiration Dates?

The FDA requires expiration dates to be printed on the packaging for drugs, including sunscreens and anti-perspirants, but not for cosmetic products. However, most cosmetic companies formulate products to have a 2-3 year shelf life. Since it's not required, most cosmetic companies have not traditionally printed the expiration date on the package - but more and more manufacturers have begun printing expiration dates on cosmetic packaging recently.

Parabens

What are they? Parabens are used in food, pharmaceuticals and cosmetics as a preservative, primarily used to extend the shelf life of products. You can find them on ingredient statements listed as: Methylparaben, Propylparaben, Ethylparaben and Butylparaben.

Why do we need any preservatives? Well, not only do preservatives extend the shelf life of a product, they also protect against microbial contamination. Imagine making a glass of ice tea. How long would you let it sit around - and still be willing to drink it? A day, a week, a year? Yuck! Okay, sorry about that image. Now, imagine a cosmetic product - especially if made with natural ingredients. Typically, the cosmetic industry formulates a product capable of withstanding a two to three year shelf life. Why so long? Some cosmetic companies suggest you dispose of any product that has been open and partially used after six months. However, most people don't realize that once a product is manufactured, it is shipped to a distribution warehouse, then to the retailer where a product can sit on a shelf from one to even several months before being purchased. Then it sits on your bathroom counter until you use it up or the six months passes.

While parabens have been the most commonly used preservative system in cosmetics, their use is becoming increasingly controversial. Parabens have been identified in biopsy samples from breast tumors and have also been found in almost all urine samples examined from a diverse sample of US adults. Parabens have been categorized as Endocrine Disruptors, which is when a synthetic chemical is absorbed into the body and mimics or blocks hormones, disrupting the body's normal functions.

How can you avoid them? Some companies have introduced products in airless containers and claim their products are preservative free. However, I have two issues with this type of claim. First, airless containers may prevent contamination after purchase, however, I believe all products should have preservatives to prevent microbial problems created from the packaging, manufacturing, warehousing of components or even the raw materials themselves. Secondly, most raw materials are shipped to a manufacturer with a preservative already in them. While it is "understood" that the raw material had to be preserved to provide shelf life, the preservative used in manufacturing the raw material may not be disclosed on the ingredient statement of the finished product – since no additional preservatives were added. In which case, the product really isn't preservative free – is it?

Maybe a safer statement may be "No Preservatives Added."

Be Informed

To be clear, I am not saying that the cosmetic claims have no merit or that no skin care product works - that's not the case at all. My intention is for you to be better informed and understand how claims are written and what can legally be said about a cosmetic product. This way, you will have a better understanding of what is actually being said - and not just misinterpret these statements for what you want to hear or understand. The key is to read each claim and each ingredient statement carefully. Remember, caveat emptor.

Is It Worth The Money?

One of the biggest questions I am asked is if the discount brands are as good as the expensive brands. Not to sound indecisive, but "Yes" and "No." I want to explain and help give you an understanding, so you can decide which is the smartest bet for you.

First, a lot of women in their twenties and thirties do not have the same disposable income as those in their forties, fifties, sixties and older. The cost of a product can be of great concern

You are already beautiful. But a basic skin care routine provides healthier-looking skin now, while helping to protect your skin against damage that will appear years from now.

Healthy skin requires work, just like a healthy body. At the absolute minimum, you need to cleanse and replenish your skin – remove makeup and impurities, following that with a moisturizer to help hydrate the skin. These steps are a must – *every day!* To me, it's like exercising, where walking even a little every day is better than no exercise at all.

So, if you are on a budget, do your research and buy the best you can get for the price. Don't put off beginning a healthy skincare regimen until you can afford the most expensive products. Using a basic, inexpensive product is better than using no product at all - as long as the product you select is made with healthy, quality ingredients.

While I often question the quality of some of the inexpensive products out there, I do believe that it is both important and possible to find quality, affordable solutions – even just the daily essentials: cleanser, daily moisturizer, and eye gel or eye cream! Just be sure to read the ingredient statement to verify that the products are free of soap-based emulsifiers and other harmful ingredients discussed in this book. For help in your shopping, visit my website www.JustAskDavid.com and download the pocket size list of the Top Ingredients To Avoid.

What About Those Expensive Products?

There is a lot that goes into the cost of a cosmetic product: retailers' profit margins, the gifts with purchase, advertising and promotional expenses, plus the cost of creating the product – including the cost of the packaging, research & development, manufacturing, the company's operational expenses, etc. What's left is available for the cost of chemicals and, of course, the company's profits. Thus, the moderate and more expensive products are able to use more expensive, higher-quality ingredients, higher actives concentrations, etc. But, "buyer beware," this isn't always the case; there's no denying that some products are just more expensive because they carry a well-perceived brand name or designer label.

Invest in quality products. Don't get caught up in the hype or the media hype. Be sure to evaluate the ingredient statements and ask the right questions to know you are getting your money's worth.

I think most people would be surprised to learn that just one full-page ad in a well-known fashion/beauty magazine can cost $130,000![1] That's right – just one page, just for the one issue. That does not include the cost of a model, the photography, or the advertising agency's creative work. Now, imagine the amount a cosmetic company spends when they place a several-page ad, in several different magazines, month after month after month. Who pays for that? Of course, the cost has to be built in to the price of the products.

While an ingredient statement can tell you what is in the product and at what approximate levels, what you don't know is the quality of the ingredients. Manufacturers can purchase a particular ingredient from a variety of suppliers, each with different quality or activity levels.

To me, it's like comparing an expensive restaurant to an inexpensive restaurant. Or, even a meal basic like steak. Steak all comes from cows, but there are different breeds (Angus, etc.), different feeds and grazing methods (grass- versus grain-fed), and different cuts (chuck versus filet mignon) – all this before a good or bad chef or restaurant even gets it into their hands. More often than not, the quality of the ingredients varies greatly.

Each company operates differently. Some will spend less on advertising or packaging – or earn a smaller profit – putting the extra money into building a better product in order to build a repeat customer. Others simply cut corners to make as much as they can, ignoring the possibility of a repeat customer.

There are some very good brands out there. So, how do you know if the product you're considering will truly work and if it's worth the money? There are several options:

1) **REVIEWS:** Read product reviews at various websites (not just the manufacturers) and blogs. Be aware, most website

software lets companies remove or control comments and reviews – and many companies write favorable online reviews of their own products. So, personally, I prefer not to rely on reviews posted on the manufacturer's website, but rather reviews posted on various retailer websites where the product is carried. A number of retailers will allow positive and negative posts made by customers.

2) **ASK A FRIEND:** Ask a friend or family member if they have ever used the product. Make sure to reciprocate. So, when you find a great product, make sure to share your news with friends and family – or add to a blog posting.

3) **SAMPLES:** Ask for a sample and evaluate the product yourself, before spending your hard-earned cash. If your retailer does not have samples, contact the manufacturer directly.

4) **GUARANTEE:** Ask the retailer about their return policy, or contact the manufacturer directly for their return policy. The easiest solution is to be able to return a product to the retailer, but you want to make sure the manufacturer believes in the product enough to stand behind it. You want to make sure that there is a satisfaction guarantee, not just a return policy for an unused product. What's the difference? A satisfaction guarantee lets you actually use the product; then, if you try it and are not satisfied with the results, you can return it for a full refund not just exchange it for another product. If a manufacturer's claims are real, if the manufacturer believes in the product, and if the manufacturer wants to earn a long-term customer, this is   a reasonable expectation on your part.

5) **REVIEW INGREDIENTS:** You don't have to be a chemist! You just learned the secret of how to read the ingredient statement to understand if the ingredients the manufacturer claims to be in your product are really there, and whether these ingredients are used at meaningful levels or just trace levels.

6) **DISSECT THE CLAIMS:** Thoroughly read the claims, look for the buzzwords and disclaimers, think about what you're really being told, and be realistic about your expectations.

~ Chapter Four ~

Is Your Skin Cream Aging You Faster Think You Think?

None of us feel our age. None of us think we look our age. None of us want to admit our age. However, your skin cream could be working against you, damaging your skin and actually making you look older – faster than you think!

It reminds me of the story where an older lady had just moved to a new city. She had needed to find a new doctor. While sitting in the waiting room on the day of her first appointment, she noticed the doctor's diploma on the wall and the doctor's full name.

She immediately recalled a boy with the same name that she had had a secret crush on some 50 years earlier. But when the doctor came out, she realized this couldn't be the same boy. The doctor was an older man with deep wrinkles on his face; he was balding and what hair was left was gray.

At the end of the appointment, she couldn't resist asking, "Doctor, can I ask where you grew up?" The lady was surprised to hear his reply, which was the same town she was from. So, she continued, "Can I ask what high school you attended?" The doctor acted very proud and announced he was a "Northern Illinois Titan! Wait. Why do you ask?"

She replied that she was, too, and that she remembered him from back in the day.

The doctor looked at her closely, and this old, wrinkled, balding, gray haired man asked her, "What did you teach?"

Obviously, we all get older - but we don't want to look older faster than we have to. In this chapter, I want to expose some of the ingredients that may be in products you use every day that may actually be doing more harm than good. In fact, a number of cosmetic and skin care products, including moisturizers, contain ingredients that actually dry the skin - leaving your skin more damaged than if no product had been used at all!

Even worse, some of the ingredients in the products you use as part of your daily beauty regimen are actually harmful to humans - and even considered by the FDA as carcinogens that may cause cancer!

Is Your Moisturizer Drying Your Skin?

Before I unlock the secrets of how certain skin care formulations can actually damage the skin and how you, too, can become an expert at which products to buy and which ones to avoid, I think it's important for you to understand a few of the basics about how our skin works.

I actually lecture on this topic at various seminars around the country. When I speak in front of a group of doctors, I see them shaking their heads in agreement - these dermatologists, plastic surgeons, or other physicians just don't understand why the cosmetic industry hasn't solved this key issue. When I speak in front of members of the beauty industry or chemists, they often admit that they would be capable of creating healthier, less damaging products – but they just simply didn't understand the negative effects that some of their most basic ingredients have on the skin.

Don't worry, there won't be a test at the end, but I think the next few pages will help you understand a few things that most people, including many experts in the cosmetic industry, just don't get.

The Basics

Our skin is the body's largest organ and does more than just keep our bodies and internal organs intact. The skin is made of three main layers, known as the Epidermis, Dermis and Hypodermis – and it serves three key functions:

1. PROTECTION: against impurities, pollutants, disease-causing agents, chemicals, the sun's harmful rays, bacterial infections, temperatures, and other external threats.

2. REGULATION: of body temperature and moisture. Temperature is controlled through both perspiration and the action of the blood vessels located in the dermis layer, which increase blood flow when hot and restrict blood flow when cold. Moisture is regulated through perspiration and the skin's lipid barrier,

which provides a semi-impermeable barrier to keep moisture in and minimize Trans-Epidermal Water Loss(TEWL).

3. PERCEPTION: of you and for you. In other words, the skin has receptors and nerve endings that allow us to feel hot, cold, rough, smooth, pain or other physical sensations; while skin firmness, wrinkles, and pigmentation affecting appearance and how you are perceived by others.

Skin Layers

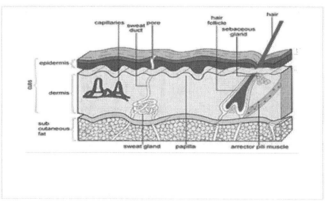

Epidermis – the outermost layer provides resistance and protection. The Epidermis is comprised of several distinct layers, beginning with the stratum corneum and ending with the basal cell layer. The Epidermis is in a constant state of renewal, with skin cells slowly working their way up to the top layer as older cells are sloughed off.

Dermis – the middle layer consists of connective tissue and provides flexible support structure (or cushion) to protect the body from stain and stress. The Dermis contains collagen, elastin, glycosaminoglycans (hyaluronic acid, chondroitin sulfate, dermatan sulfate), and also blood vessels, nerve endings, sweat glands, hair follicles and sebaceous glands. Since collagen and elastin are synthesized in the Dermis, this is the targeted area in some of the recent breakthroughs in skin care.

Hypodermis (*subcutaneous adipose layer*) – contains the adipose tissue (subcutaneous fat) and provides a thermal barrier and mechanical cushion ("padding"), in addition to attaching the dermis to the underlying tissues. The Hypodermis contains 50% of our body fat.

While our skin has three key layers, our primary focus is going to be on the Epidermis – the outermost layer. The Epidermis is often described as a sort of wall, made of brick and mortar, with the inactive skin cells being the bricks and the skin's lipid matrix being the mortar – or glue – that holds them together. Together, they make up our body's most important protective barrier.

Is Your Skin Care Actually Aging You?

The sad irony is that, while our skin works very hard to protect us, we don't do a very good job of taking care of our skin –

even when we think we are. The skin care we use every day may actually be harming our skin and accelerating the signs of aging.

Traditional Skin Cream Formula:

60 – 90%   Water and water-soluble ingredients

5 – 25%   Emollients, oils and oil-soluble ingredients

5 – 15%   Soap-based binding ingredients, called emulsifiers

Back in elementary school, we were all taught that oil and water do not mix. Well – in foods and cosmetics – we make them mix. To bring them together and bind them, chemists use what are called emulsifiers. Emulsifiers are typically soap-based binding ingredients that hold the ingredients together. Without emulsifiers, your cosmetic creams and lotions would separate and you would constantly be stirring or shaking them in an attempt to mix the two together, like Italian salad dressings where the oil and vinegar separate.

Here's the problem with using these soap-based emulsifiers. When you apply a skin cream, the water and water-soluble ingredients are either absorbed or evaporate, while the emollients and oils are absorbed. What remains on the surface of the skin is the soap-based emulsifier residue, which stays there until you wash it off. And this soap residue can actually damage your skin.

Fun Experiment

Take a large dinner plate or wide bowl. Pour in some tap water. Sprinkle ground black pepper on top of the water. Next, put liquid dishwashing soap on your finger tip. Place your finger on the edge of the water and watch the pepper.

Explanation: Water molecules are "polar," meaning that water molecules have a positive region and a negative region – reversing their orientation, as necessary, to join together. The water bond or cluster creates surface tension, allowing some items to float. Soap, however, varies and has either a positive or negative charge – so water loves to bond to soap, breaking the surface tension of the water. Where there is no soap, surface tension remains strong and the pepper floats. However, as soap is added, the strong water bonds move away from the soap, carrying the pepper with it – creating the illusion of the pepper "running away."

In skin care, we want to combine oil-soluble ingredients and water-soluble ingredients. Oil is non-polar and does not combine with the water molecules directly. However, soap molecules reduce the water's surface tension and create mutual bond between the water and the oil. The soap is the binding agent, or emulsifier.

So, unfortunately, while some of the active ingredients in the product you just applied may have a beneficial effect, these effects are minimized or even completely reversed by the damage caused by the soap residue that the emulsifier left behind. And here's the really important part: *every cream or lotion you use contains an emulsifier or emulsifiers.* But why, again, is this a problem?

The answer is because soap residue damages skin in 3 ways:

1. **DISRUPTS pH** - The top layers of our skin are actually acidic, creating an acid mantle to provide antimicrobial protection, as well as promoting normal skin homeostasis (or normal skin renewal). Our skin's normal pH ranges from 4.5 to 5.3, a number which varies from person to person – starting low and increasing with age. However, the majority of skin care products have a pH of 6 to 7 (in the slightly more alkaline range). This pH level helps manufacturers' products minimize irritation and helps to improve formulation stability. However, while this is beneficial to the manufacturer, it is not beneficial to you.

   The soap residue left on the skin disrupts and perpetuates this abnormal pH until you wash it away. That means that when you put on your favorite moisturizer or foundation, you are actually disrupting your skin's normal process – all day long. In an effort to fight back, your body produces excess oils (or sebum). This pH war creates different skin types and results in problems like rosacea, adult acne, and the premature signs of aging.

Some manufacturers have introduced products with lower pH levels. Unfortunately, that is not enough to keep our skin healthy and repairing itself. Remember, each of us has a unique pH. So, while selecting a product with a lower pH may help, that alone does not go far enough. The real answer is to find products that do not leave behind a soap-based residue and do not interfere with our individual pH. Emerging technologies are beginning to answer these needs, allowing products to be effective without damaging the skin. We will discuss these in more depth shortly.

2. **IMPEDES SKIN HEALING** – While scientists have long known that the skin's surface is acidic, it has only been in the past few years that they have discovered that, when the skin's pH is normal, it produces enzymes that trigger the formation of essential lipids and actually repair the skin's protective barrier – a process called homeostasis. However, when our normal pH is disrupted, so is the skin's renewal process.

3. **DAMAGES THE LIPID BARRIER** – Soap residue slowly attacks and emulsifies the lipids (healthy fats) in our skin throughout the day. Then, upon washing, these emulsified skin lipids are actually rinsed away with the soap residue, removing an important part of our protective barrier. This works in much the same way that the soap-based emulsifier was used to help bind the water- and oil-based ingredients and carry them into your skin; the soap now binds with your

skin's natural oils and carries them out – leaving your skin drier than before. You've felt these effects in more obvious ways, for example, that is what you're experiencing when your hands or face feel dry and tight after being washed with soap. The resulting damage can lead to drier skin, accelerate the signs of aging, and cause other skin ailments.

Is There An Alternative?

Bottom line: the soap-based emulsifiers used in the majority of skin care creams and cosmetic foundations actually damage the skin and, at the end of the day, leave the skin drier than if no skin care product was used at all. And you paid for the privilege!

So, what can you do to treat your skin well? One solution is to apply a moisturizer twice a day, which is what the cosmetic companies prefer. However, you would still be robbing your skin of moisture as a result of the soap-based emulsifiers – but at least you would be replenishing some of that lost moisture more frequently.

But what about a better solution? Can you imagine if your skin cream didn't create this damage in the first place? Can't the cosmetics industry develop new technologies and create new, healthier products that don't contain soap-based emulsifiers? Well, **the good news is that these products now exist!** Instead of requiring the use of an additional moisturizer at night just to maintain skin hydration, new trends in *soap-free emulsifiers* will actually help beauty products increase the level of skin hydration – and without the damage! These products aren't yet widespread, but, as cosmetic companies learn more, *and as women demand* *healthier products*, the industry will be forced to respond. You can be a part of this positive change by writing to your favorite cosmetic companies or by simply "voting with your pocketbook" – that is, purchasing products that already use this emerging soap-free emulsification technology. For the most up to date information, visit my website at **www.JustAskDavid.com.**

How Can You Tell?

How can you tell if your favorite products contain soap-based emulsifiers? Let me help! Take a moment. Go get your favorite skin creams, body lotions, cosmetic foundations, etc. Read the labels. Typically, these ingredients will be found halfway through the list or closer to the end. These harmful soap-based emulsifiers will be listed under a variety of different names. Some ingredient listings may contain an additional word or number, but you can easily spot them by looking for ingredients containing the word or words:

"Emulsifying Wax," "Polysorbate," "Stearate," "Steareth," "Cetearyl," "Ceteareth," and many others. *(For a more complete list, visit my website* **www.JustAskDavid.com** *and look in our resource section.)*

~ Chapter Five ~

Does Your Skin Cream Cause Cancer?

BUT WAIT...
How Could It Get Even Worse?

DOES Your Favorite Skin Cream

Cause CANCER?

1,4-Dioxane

While we have discussed the damage caused by soap-based emulsifiers, the real truth about their use in your skin-care products is even worse. That's because, to make these soap-based emulsifiers, the emulsifiers undergo a chemical process called "ethoxylation."

Ethoxylation is a process of adding ethylene oxide, a known carcinogen, to create a less harsh ingredient. This process generates a byproduct called 1,4-Dioxane. You won't find this ingredient on the ingredient listing, since the FDA does not require the listing of a byproduct – but it is still present in the f inal product. In a moment, I will tell you how to determine if it is in your favorite personal care products.

1,4-Dioxane is a hidden contaminant found in a number of shampoos, body washes – even baby shampoos and bubble baths. 1,4-Dioxane is considered a human carcinogen by the U.S. Environmental Protection Agency (EPA) and the U.S. Food and Drug Administration (FDA). In addition, it is included in California's Proposition 65 list of chemicals known or suspected to cause cancer or birth defects.

Since 1979, the FDA has been measuring 1,4-Dioxane levels. While the FDA has followed up on skin absorption studies that showed that 1,4-Dioxane can penetrate the skin when applied in certain preparations (like lotions). The FDA has determined that, due to the low levels of 1,4-Dioxane typically found in cosmetics, and because they only remain, on the skin for only several hours, there is not a significant danger to consumers.

Even so, in 2000, the FDA recommended that cosmetic products should voluntarily reduce the level of 1,4-Dioxane to no more than 10 parts-per-million. The FDA does not test cosmetics for safety before they are introduced to the market. It is up to individual cosmetic manufacturers to choose to adopt the FDA's recommendations, but it is not required – and there are reports of well-known brands with levels exceeding the FDA guidelines.

Even if each product you use does meet the guidelines, there is another problem. Do you use only one product each day? The question must be raised:

"What is the hazard to consumers if repeated exposure occurs through the use non-compliant products or the use of multiple products at the same time? And do you really want to be exposed to ANY level of a known carcinogen?"

Does Your Skin Cream Cause Cancer?

While shampoos and body washes have recently gained attention in the media for the presence of 1,4-Dioxane, no one has yet talked about the ethoxylated emulsifiers used in skin creams. That's right. The majority of skin creams, lotions, foundations, and other topically-applied emulsions contain 1,4-Dioxane.

So let's take another look at your favorite personal care products. Review the ingredient statements again, this time looking for ingredients that contain 1,4-Dioxane. According to the FDA, ethoxylated chemicals containing 1,4-Dioxane can be identified by the following prefix, word, or syllables:

> "PEG," "Polyethylene," "Polyethylene Glycol," "Polyoxyethylene," or ending with "-oxynol' or '-eth" (such as Ceteareth or others)

STOP! Take a look at your current skin care products. Does your current skin cream cause cancer?

What Are The Alternatives?

For shampoos and body washes, the answer for consumers is simple – avoid those with ethoxylated ingredients. For manufacturers, the solution is to develop and use ingredients and processes that don't produce 1,4-Dioxane. Unfortunately, some manufacturers have resisted the change because of the associated costs. Another solution is for raw material producers, themselves, to remove the 1,4-Dioxane byproduct through a process called "vacuum stripping," before shipping the active ingredients to the manufacturers and big cosmetic brands. Again, there are associated costs involved.

I know this change can be done. How do I know? Because healthy ingredients and production practices are already being used overseas. In fact, numerous countries, including those in the European Union, have strict guidelines regulating which ingredients are safe and can be used.

> **And here's the part that should make you really angry** – Some multi-national companies actually use different formulations for the products they distribute in the U.S. and those they distribute to Europe. That means that they use ethoxylated ingredients in the United States and safer, non-ethoxylated versions in other countries. That's right, some U.S.-based companies continue to use the ethoxylated materials, which contain known cancer-causing ingredients, in their own backyard, while using non-ethoxylated formulations overseas.

For skin care creams and lotions, the answer is not as simple. The problem is that no one has really talked about 1,4-Dioxane in skin creams. The focus has, instead, been on products like body washes and shampoos. So, one of my goals with this book is to build awareness of this un-publicized concern. I need your help, but, together, we can make a difference.

What can you do? You can make a difference by letting manufacturers and retailers know it matters to you by a) reading labels and purchasing brands that have already taken the responsible step to use non-ethoxylated ingredients or b) writing to manufacturers and retailers to let them know how you feel. If consumers start speaking out, manufacturers will be forced to make the change!

Some raw material suppliers have already listened and started working on alternatives. And safer options, like those used in Europe, already exist. But truly responsible chemists and companies are starting to experiment with entirely new types of delivery systems and new methods of formulating products. The race is on to develop emulsification alternatives that are *soap-free,* as well as 1,4-Dioxane free.

As the authority in the beauty industry and someone who is "standing on his soap box" and letting consumers and the world know about this problem, you can see why some companies are racing to meet with me to discuss how to adapt their product lines. However, there are others that would prefer that the message never got out. I have had some people point out that if the cosmetic companies acknowledge the problem, take a proactive stance, and promote a new method of formulating; it could actually damage the credibility and sales of all their other products. They would, in effect, be admitting there is and has been a problem – and that they've knowingly been selling harmful products to U.S. consumers. I understand the dilemma, but believe that the industry, as a whole, must make take a long view and make a positive change – for the sake of the industry, for the sake of the consumer, and for the sake of doing the right thing!

SMART Core™ Science

I have combined my experience as a cosmetic chemist, the authority in beauty, and a consumer advocate, to help form a company focused on developing a revolutionary new emulsion system that is soap-free and enhances the delivery of key ingredients. We threw out traditional production methods and took a totally new approach, by working synergistically with the body. The end result is SMART Core™ science.

Inspired by two-time Nobel Prize winner Dr. Linus Pauling, SMART Core™ science solves the problems associated with soap-based skin creams.

Normally, H_2O (water) molecules attract each other and "associate" themselves randomly, creating a disordered, chaotic cluster. These unorganized clusters can easily bond with impurities and have a negative effect on the skin.

SMARTCore™ science solves this problem by employing a unique energizing process that organizes and structures smaller H_2O clusters, enhancing the absorption through cell walls. The energized and structured H_2O molecules are then linked with Phospholipids, Triglycerides, Ceramides, and Cholesterol to mimic the skin's own protective barrier.

SMART Core™ end result is a new generation of skin care that does not use soap-based emulsifiers and is clinically proven to increase skin hydration...all day long!

SMART Core™ benefits:

- Soap & Surfactant Free
- Self-Adjusts To Skin's Natural pH
- Time-Release Delivery Of Active Ingredients
- Promotes Natural Skin Repair
- Maximizes Skin Hydration
- Creates The Next Generation In Skin Care

This is one of the most important breakthroughs in the Science of Beauty! And this technology is already being used in a number of skin care products. To find products based on SMART Core™, look for the logo on the package or ask the cosmetic manufacturer if they are using SMART Core™.

For more information, visit:

www.SMARTCoreScience.com

Going Beyond Green – Going Safe

Today's consumer is more health conscious and more environmentally conscious, and she understands the importance of "going green." But being a responsible and educated consumer goes beyond that. Consumers are becoming more and more aware of the effects of toxic chemicals on our bodies and the earth.

Currently, the U.S. has banned or restricted only 11 ingredients for use in cosmetics, while, in the European countries, the EU Cosmetics Directive bans or restricts 1,100 ingredients found to be harmful. Some multi-national companies have simply created one set of products for the United States and another for the rest of the world.

The body's largest organ is our skin. Up to 60% of certain ingredients found in our personal care products, including face moisturizers, body lotions, and bath gels, will absorb into our skin and end up in the bloodstream, according to a CBS News Report. These chemicals can accumulate in target organs or be metabolized through our system, sometimes over a period of years, according to Mount Sinai.

Natural Solutions magazine, in collaboration with the national retailer Whole Foods, ranked the top dangerous chemicals found in personal care products. This list includes Parabens, Polyethylene Glycol (PEG), Sodium Lauryl/Laureth Sulfates, Petrochemicals like Mineral Oil and Petrolatum, Synthetic Fragrances, and Synthetic Colorants. Side effects from these harmful chemicals are reported to include hormone disruption, hampering the skin's ability to breathe, clogging pores, causing skin rashes and eye irritation, damaging the reproductive system, and others. Some retailers are creating new standards for products they carry, disallowing ethoxylation, and requiring many companies to reformulate and replace ingredients known to be associated with 1,4-Dioxane.

In an effort to protect the health of consumers and workers, by securing the corporate, regulatory, and legislative reforms necessary to eliminate dangerous chemicals from cosmetics and personal care products, the Campaign for Safe Cosmetics was formed. The Campaign for Safe Cosmetics is working with more than 100 endorsing organizations, thousands of grassroots supporters, and over 1,300 U.S. companies that have signed the "Compact for Safe Cosmetics" and are leading the way in innovating safer products.

Before you buy your next product, look to see if your favorite cosmetic company has signed the Compact for Safe Cosmetics. In addition, the Environmental Working Group (EWG) has established "Skin Deep" – a cosmetics database that acts as your safety guide to cosmetics and personal care products. You can look up your favorite products, their ingredient statements, or even particular ingredients to find out the safety score. Visit **www.JustAskDavid.com** for links to these sites and other resources.

Conclusion

I hate to say it, but you have reached the end of the book. I hope you have enjoyed reading it, even half as much as I have enjoyed writing it! As the authority in beauty, I have seen a lot and as a consumer advocate, my goal was to share some of the secrets of the beauty industry and empower you to be able to make the decisions that are right for you.

In addition to enjoying a few humorous stories, I hope you learned:

1. That YOU ARE beautiful – just the way you are! While the fashion and beauty magazines try to set an unrealistic standard of beauty, the truth is everyone sees something different – making each of us beautiful just as we are, in our own way.

2. What you eat can impact your skin – from the inside, out. Some foods supply essential nutrients, while others can help with specific needs – and others can actually counteract the benefits of your beauty regimen. Simple adjustments in your daily routine can make an incredible impact on the overall health of your skin and your glowing, youthful appearance.

3. The TRUTH about what's really inside your favorite beauty products, how to better understand the advertising and product claims made by manufacturers, and the tricks the beauty industry plays to make products sound better.

4. Which ingredients can damage your skin and even accelerate the signs of aging. The new frontier in skin care is not natural ingredients, but rather *Safe Cosmetics* that avoid ingredients that are dangerous to our health.

5. How to review the ingredient statement to determine if the product contains the hidden cancer causing ingredient 1,4-Dioxane and what safe alternatives are available.

I invite you to share this book with your friends and family. I also invite you to visit my on-line magazine www.JustAskDavid.com for the latest information, to access additional resources, share how this book has helped you, and even submit any questions you may have. I look forward to hearing from you!

THANK YOU!

The Authority in Beauty
David Pollock

Remember – have a question?
Do what the big brands do,

Just Ask David!